Putting the Pieces Together

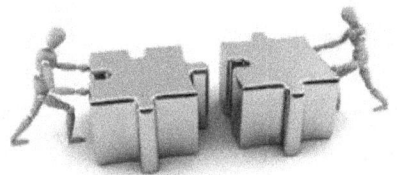

For a Longer, Heathier Life

Healthy Aging – Putting it all Together

L J Samuels

Contents

Fred Astaire is reported to have said,

'Old age is like everything else. To make a success of it, you've got to start young.'

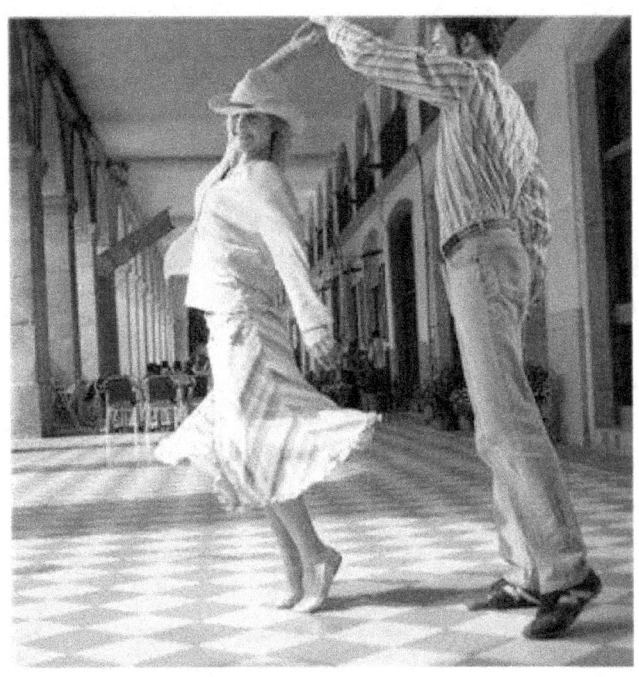

Healthy Aging – Putting it all Together

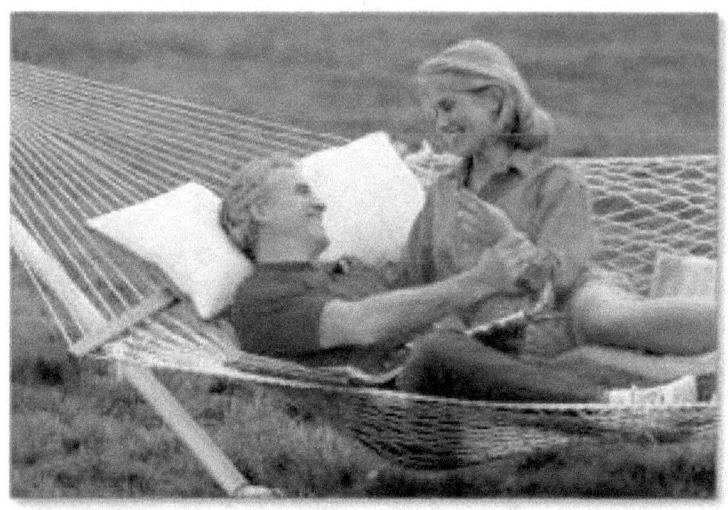

Introduction

I really am not an exercise and fitness fanatic but as I got older I realised that, although my brain was still fully functioning, my body was showing signs of slowing down.

It had started to produce those little aches and pains – you know the type; when you get up from the chair it takes a few steps before your feet allow you to walk normally.

I sometimes found myself making the 'umpff' noise when getting up from the chair or picking something up off the floor.

Even though I had taken reasonable care of myself I knew that I could do more. So I decided that it was time to make sure that, as I continue to get older, I was as fit and healthy as I could possibly be. I decided that it was time to make the effort to eat healthily and exercise regularly so I could make the most of my life.

Now I don't know about you, but when I did any exercise I invariably came home feeling invigorated and good about myself. .

Whatever type of exercise you do; walking the dog, using the treadmill, going to the gym, even just getting off the bus a few stops earlier than normal can make you feel good about yourself.

In fact, any activity that increases the heart rate even slightly will help to produce the 'happy hormones'.

These hormones are really called endorphins – but I just like the vision that the words 'happy hormones' bring to mind. You know, two yellow smiley faces holding hands and dancing around.

From the age of 35 changes begin to take place in the average person's body. Muscle mass reduces, muscle elasticity reduces, bone density declines, the metabolism slows down whilst body fat increases.

But there are steps you can take to minimise the effect that these declines could have on your life and the aim of this book is to lead you in the right direction.

I have also included 25 Health and Fitness Facts as well as some quick, easy and healthy recipes that are easily adaptable to your own personal taste.

I hope you get some benefit from reading this book and commit yourself to improving your chances of having a long and, more importantly, healthy life.

Interesting Fact:

Recently there has been research completed that shows aerobic exercise (any exercise that increases respiration and heart rates) can actually help slow down the memory loss process which inevitably happens as we age.

Problems with Weight Gain as you Age

As you get older, your body's metabolism starts naturally slowing down. Add to this the fact that most people over 45 are usually more sedentary than in their earlier years, and in a lot of cases, you have weight gain.

Being over 45 and trying to get fit and lose weight is more challenging than it was when you were in your twenties and thirties, but that doesn't mean it's too hard to do.

You don't need to deny yourself anything or go on a crash diet; with the *right* diet and exercise you can be healthier and happier than ever before.

Modern Lifestyle

How many of us can honestly say that we get enough exercise? It may be that we feel we can't find the time or when we finish work, we are simply too tired to get out there and make the effort.

Did you know that exercise can increase the levels of our 'happy hormone'? It is the endorphins that are manufactured in our brain that make us feel good after we have exercised. So, if you find yourself using any excuse to avoid exercising, remember the 'happy hormone' and how good you will feel after you've been for a run, a brisk walk or even a gentle swim.

We were never designed to live the sedentary lifestyle that today's world has forced upon us.

Why Should We Exercise?

In caveman times, when we were hunter gathers, we would have had to walk for miles to find our lunch. Then we would have had to carry it back to the cave (or where-ever), cleaned and cooked it (I think) before we could sit down to dine.

We would have done the same thing all over again the day after. So, getting enough exercise was never an issue, it would have been necessary to keep ourselves alive.

Oh, I know that those days are long gone - thankfully.

But our body design remains fundamentally the same and the effect of sitting around in an office and the convenience lifestyle that we have adopted, is now beginning to take its toll.

So, in order to become as healthy as we can possibly be, we have to design our modern lifestyle around exercise and a healthy diet.

Research suggests that today's obesity problems are possibly caused more by lack of exercise rather than consistently over eating. Being a couch potato, coupled with the wrong type of diet, would cause anyone to gain some extra pounds.

So, it is in our best interests to combine regular exercise with a healthy diet which will help to ensure that we will be around to see our grandchildren grow up.

Exercise alone is not the answer, nor is diet, but both together can make a big difference to our overall health and could also help to increase our life expectancy.

Possible Causes of Weight Gain in Older People

Menopause

As women and men age, their metabolism changes. One of the main causes of this in women is menopause. The oestrogen levels drop off and women will experience many changes, including possible weight gain. Because of the decline in oestrogen and other changes in the body, we start to eat different things. This is because the body may not be able to digest things as well as it did before.

If digestion is impeded, then we may not get the "I'm full" signal as quickly as we did before.

Another reason for the change in the things we eat is that our taste buds are not as sensitive as they used to be and we need more, and different, flavours to make our food enjoyable.

Stress

Beginning at around the age of 40-45 and continuing, men and women produce more of the stress hormone cortisol. As cortisol production increases, so does your belly fat. Gaining weight around your middle is going to be the most difficult place to lose it.

In addition to naturally producing more cortisol, you may be experiencing profound life changes. Impending retirement, empty nest syndrome, worry about aging, and an ever changing body image can cause stress.

Lack of Sleep

For both men and women over 45, insomnia is common. This is because the sleep hormone melatonin is not released in the higher levels it used to be. Part of the reason for this is the increased level of cortisol.

This causes a domino effect. You have no energy, you're in a bad mood, and it gets more and more difficult to motivate yourself to move. (Later in this book I will give you more information on how to improve your mood and motivation).

All of these things lead to a more sedentary lifestyle – but only if you allow it to happen.

Menopause causes hormone levels to fluctuate, causing you to eat more. Cortisol production increases and melatonin production decreases, causing you to lose sleep.

Result: Lack of sleep leaves you with no energy or desire to get up and exercise.

Loss of Muscle Mass

As you age it becomes more difficult to maintain muscle mass. Muscles burn more calories than fat, so when you start losing muscle mass, your metabolism slows down.

A reduction in calories along with an appropriate exercise program will help keep your weight in check.

Health Concerns

The state of your health at 40 and over can mean the difference between an active lifestyle in your advancing years and a life of worry and stress.

If you do not maintain a reasonable level of physical fitness through diet and exercise, you are at a higher risk of developing a number of health issues including:

- Heart disease
- Diabetes
- Stroke
- Osteoporosis
- Hypertension
- Prostate Cancer
- High Cholesterol

Physical Fitness

Watching your weight and toning muscles is the key to keeping yourself healthy. Older adults who are inactive are said to be twice as likely to develop Alzheimer's disease.

Physical activity does not have to be strenuous, but it should be a regular part of your life. Being physically healthy will also give you the ability to enjoy life by being able to travel, play with your grandchildren, and take up new hobbies you'd never considered before. In fact, being physically healthy could help you work your way through your own personal 'bucket list'.

Interesting Fact:

Exercise is shown to improve cognitive function and lower depression levels. One study put exercise up against anti-depressants and found that after 16 weeks, both groups had identical improvements in mood.

This suggests that the simple act of exercising could even take the place of anti-depressant medications.

For women going through menopause, exercise could help lower the number of hot flashes and could lessen irritability.

Before you start any exercise program you may want to see your doctor to discuss it with him. This is especially true if you already have certain diseases or risk factors that physical activity may trigger.

Exercise Health and Fitness

Reminder: Please check with your doctor before embarking on any new exercise program to ensure there are no contra-indications.

Walking

Walking is the simplest form of low-impact exercise that almost everyone can do. You don't need fancy equipment, just put on a pair of comfortable shoes and walk out your front door. Take the dog; if you haven't got a dog, take your neighbour's dog, or take your neighbour…

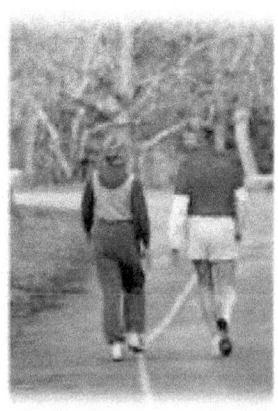

Walking is safe, doesn't require practice, and has a number of different health benefits.

- Reduces LDL cholesterol ("bad" cholesterol).
- Increases HDL cholesterol ("good" cholesterol).
- Elevates your mood (happy hormones).
- Lowers your blood pressure.
- Easy weight management technique.

When you start walking, pay attention to what you're wearing. Clothing should be comfortable and appropriate for the weather.

If you're going to walk at night, be sure to wear reflective tape and bright colours so motorists can see you.

Before you head out at full speed, you should warm up by walking at your normal walking speed for about 5 minutes to ease your muscles into activity.

After that, you need to gently stretch all of your major muscle groups.

Set small goals for yourself and slowly work up to longer distances on more days of the week. Large goals that you cannot realistically meet immediately will only discourage you.

Once you are walking your usual distance easily without breathing hard you could try fitting a few 30 second 'power walk' intervals into your walk.
Increase your speed until you are nearly jogging but don't break into a run. Simply walk very fast – go on, wiggle that behind…

Jogging

After you've been walking for a while and have got your endurance and speed to a good level, jogging is the next logical step.

Jogging is a fairly high-impact exercise. For people with no joint conditions, it is safe and will actually lower the risk of osteoporosis and increase your bone density.

Other benefits of jogging include:

- A very efficient workout that burns a lot of calories in a short amount of time.
- Your cardiovascular system will improve because the lungs and heart are forced to work harder.
- More muscle groups are engaged when you're jogging than when walking so you will lose weight and gain muscle in more areas.

If you've never jogged before, start with walking to build up your endurance.

Once you're comfortable walking and power walking for a good distance and time, start jogging in 30 second intervals during your walk. Increase that over several weeks and before you know it, you'll be jogging all the time.

Interesting Fact:

Recent research has shown that by regularly exercising for around 45 minutes, three times a week could significantly increase your life expectancy.

Running

It's never too late to begin running, as long as you are in general good health.

If you're over 50 years old you should have a health check to ensure that there are no underlying problems that could be exacerbated by taking up running.

If you have never tried running before it may be a good idea to begin with interval training. This involves fast walking for 100m then jogging for 100m for the entire time you are out and will really help to improve your stamina.

It is always good to have a running partner so you can help motivate each other.

Choose someone of similar capabilities to yourself so you can progress together.

Remember to ALWAYS warm up carefully before starting running and always stretch afterwards (warming down) to help minimise any strains.

Interesting Fact:

Did you know that more than half of the runners in the New York City Marathon are over 40 years of age?

Could this be you next year?

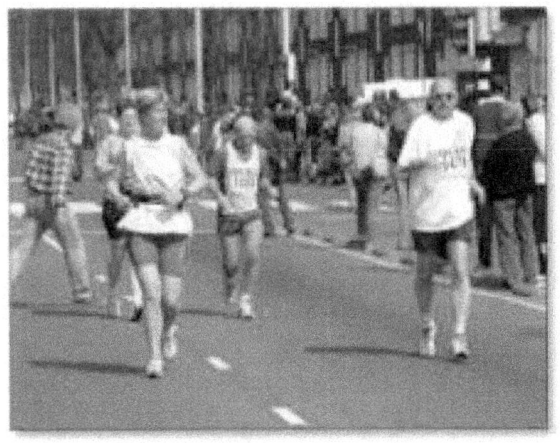

Yoga

Yoga is an ancient Hindu discipline that promotes control of both the mind and body. As you move through the poses, your stress level is reduced, your muscles are strengthened, and your flexibility and balance improves.

There are many yoga classes available for everyone, from children to seniors and includes all fitness levels.

Yoga has many benefits:

- Improved quality and quantity of sleep.
- More strength and flexibility in arthritis patients.
- Lower fasting blood sugar levels in diabetics.
- Reduction in blood pressure, cholesterol, blood sugar, and triglycerides.
- Aids in weight loss.
- Chronic pain is reduced.
- Lowered anxiety and stress levels.

You can find yoga classes at your local YMCA, college, or gym. These classes are tailored to your age group and props can be used, if you choose, to help you achieve the poses and get the most benefit from the classes.

Swimming

Swimming is a low-impact form of exercise that will increase your muscle mass, increase heart and lung function, and improve your mood. Swimming is an ideal exercise for people with asthma.

It will also give you a sense of well-being, reduce back pain or arthritis pain, and help you remain active as you age.

Start by getting a comfortable swimsuit, goggles, and possibly a swim cap if you have long hair.

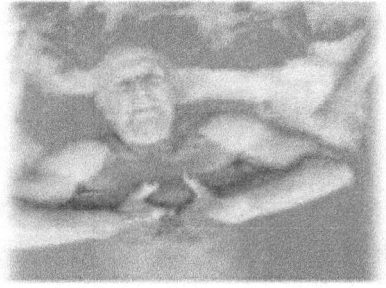

Get into the shallow end of the pool and walk to where you are the most comfortable.

Swim one lap across the pool, rest to catch your breath if you need to, and swim back.

As your lungs and muscles get used to the workout, you can add laps and speed.

Join an Aqua Aerobics session if there is one available in your area. It is fun to exercise with others and, if you find swimming laps of the pool difficult, the aqua aerobic sessions will help improve your endurance without putting any strain on your joints.

Join a Gym

Joining a gym is a great idea for you if you want to go about your exercise program under the watchful eye of a professional or using the most state of the art equipment.

Gyms often have special offers so you and a friend can sign up at a reduced cost. Working out with friends is one of the best ways to commit to an exercise program. You motivate each other to keep going through encouragement, support, and possibly a little healthy competition.

When you look for a gym to join, go in and take a tour of the facilities to make sure they have the equipment you want and that the gym is well cared for and clean.

Ask questions while you're taking the tour. Don't be shy about inquiring about anything that pops into your head. If it will make you more comfortable to have a piece of knowledge, then get it.

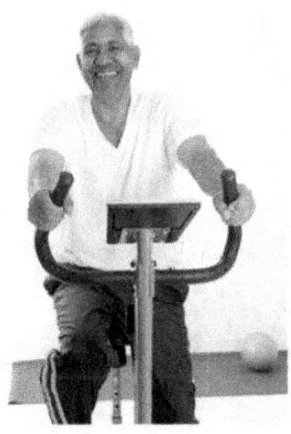

After you've chosen a gym, set up a meeting with a personal trainer. They will take your measurements and assess your strengths and weaknesses.

With that information a safe fitness plan can be developed. The fitness plan will give you realistic weekly and monthly goals to achieve. Achieving those goals will keep you motivated to keep going back.

Make sure that you communicate with the staff at the gym that you attend to keep your fitness plan up to date as you progress. They will adapt your personal plan to your current fitness levels. Having new goals to work towards will help keep you motivated.

Many gyms have special classes aimed at 'seniors'.

There could be 'spinning' classes, yoga, step classes etc. People who regularly attend these classes often form long lasting friendships with other attendees.

So this is a great way to meet like-minded people who motivate each other. Ask at your gym to see what type of classes they have to offer.

Dancing

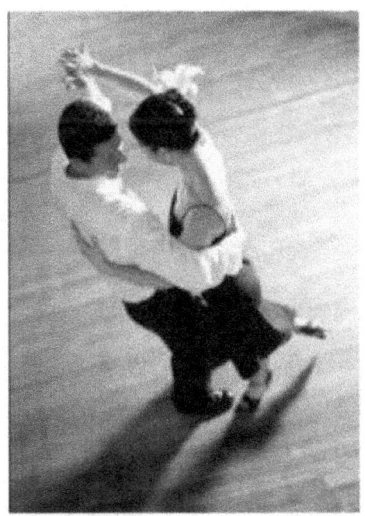

If you don't fancy any structured 'keep fit' classes try asking around to find out where you can join a dance class.

It could be Salsa, tap, ballroom dancing, line dancing etc.

Any one of these will help towards your new fitness regime whilst having a lot of fun.

You will also meet lots of new people, keep mobile and increase your fitness level whilst learning a new skill.

Make Exercise FUN

If you are not the type of person who enjoys going to the gym or getting out and about walking, running or cycling, why not try some fun activities that can involve lots of people and lots of laughs.

Remember when you were a child; did you have a skipping rope? Get one now and start skipping. Get a rope washing line and get one strong person at either end 'turning' the rope. The children will love to watch the 'oldies' skipping…

What about a hula-hoop, football, basketball, tennis racket, table tennis bat, cricket bat, badminton racket?

Are these things still in your attic gathering dust?

All these things could be reintroduced into your life to make your new fitness regime more fun. You can involve family and friends.

Have at least one day a week where you get together with a few others – maybe in your local community centre, and have some fun reintroducing a few elements of your childhood back into your life.

Start your own club and just have FUN.

Laughter is a great stress reliever and, from my own experience, there is nothing funnier than me trying to prove that I was once awesome at hula-hoop.

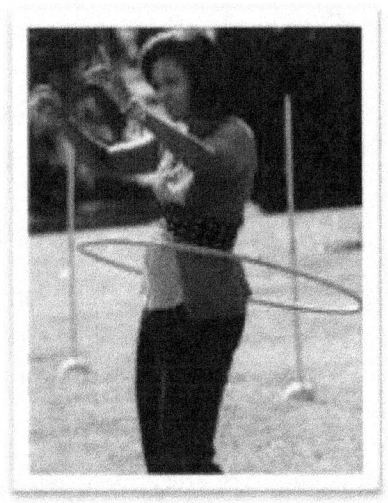

If Michelle Obama can do it...

Some Simple Exercise Solutions for Those with Reduced Mobility

There are times when the common exercises aren't an option. Some people deal with balance problems while others may not have the ability to stand in order to do the popular exercise routines that most people adopt for their healthy programs.

That doesn't mean you can't benefit from exercise. There are many sit down exercises that can help people who aren't able to stand up and move.

Here are some sit down exercises that work:

Leg extensions - Keep your feet flat on the floor. Raise one leg up until you get it as straight as you can and hold it there for a few seconds. If you can, flex your foot up while you raise the leg. These are good for your thigh and calf muscles. Repeat with the other leg. Do this exercise in a slow and controlled motion. Don't rush it.

Inner thigh exercise - Place a small object like a drinking water bottle between your inner thighs; bring your inner thighs in to gently squeeze the bottle. These are good for your inner and outer thigh muscles.

Hip flexion - Sit in a chair with your feet planted firmly on the floor (or on the foot rests of a wheelchair, if you're wheelchair-bound). Raise one leg up - keeping your knee bent and foot down. Raise the leg up a couple of inches and hold it there for a few seconds. This is good for your hip muscles.

Front raise for arms - Sit as straight as you can in a chair. Hold a drinking water bottle in one hand for a little extra added weight if you choose. With that arm straight out in front of you, raise it up shoulder level. Hold it there a little bit and release. If you choose, you can raise the arm higher as if you were raising your hand in the classroom. Repeat with the other arm.

Bicep curls - You can use the same drinking water bottle and raise your arm out to your side so that it's shoulder level. Slowly bend your elbow in, bringing the water bottle towards you as if you were doing bicep curls in a gym. Do a few repetitions with that arm and then switch to the other arm.

Abdominal exercise - Sit on the edge of your chair as straight as you can with your feet firmly planted on the floor. Raise your arms out straight in front of you and slowly lean back toward the back of the chair. When you get as far back as you can, slowly raise yourself back to a normal sitting position. Keep your abdominal muscles pulled in while you do these exercises.

Interesting Fact:

A series of 12 large scale studies found a direct link between the amount of energy a person had and the amount of physical activity they did. So if you're experiencing a slump, a 15 minute walk will do you more good than a cup of coffee or energy drink.

Changes in Diet

The number of calories the body needs reduces as your age increases.

In fact, your calorie requirement may decrease as much as 20% between the ages of 20 and 60. This is one of the main reasons that you hear people saying "It's not as easy to lose the weight these days as it was when I was in my twenties"

Women over age 45 need an average of 1800 calories a day, while men in the same age group need an average of about 2200.

Of course, this is just a generalisation as everyone is different and metabolises food at different rates. So, you should look at the calorie requirements as a guide rather than a rule.

Getting the right nutrients for a healthy mind and body is vital. To help keep your brain healthy and your mind sharp, you need to eat foods rich in omega-3 fatty acids.

Additionally, brightly coloured fruits and dark green leafy vegetables encourage brain health by improving focus and may even lower your risk of developing Alzheimer's disease.

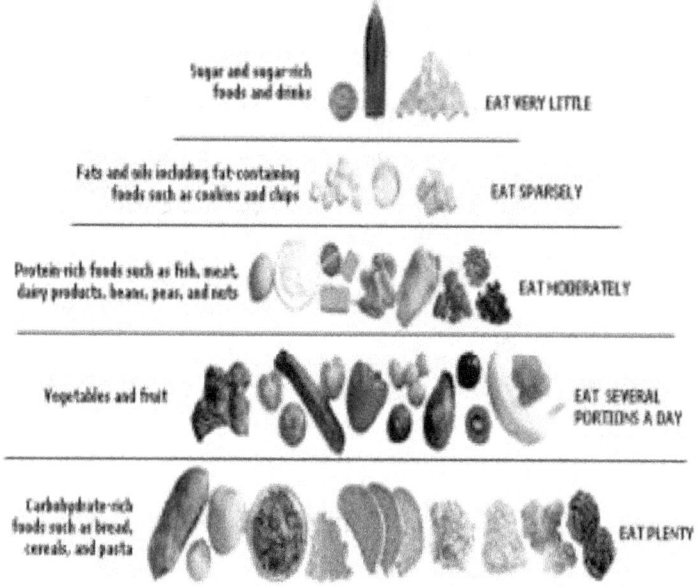

The Food Pyramid

The bulk of your healthy diet should consist of foods near the base of the pyramid: carbohydrate-rich foods, vegetables, and fruit. These supply energy, fibre, vitamins, and minerals. Protein-rich foods, in the middle row, should be eaten in moderate amounts.

Foods at the top of the pyramid, which supply energy but are low in most nutrients, are best eaten only in small amounts.

Eat Foods your Body needs

According to the Mayo Clinic, a healthy diet consists of lean protein, whole grains, fruits and vegetables. Foods high in saturated fat and cholesterol should be the exception to your eating habits, not the rule.

High fibre may aid in lowering cholesterol and omega-3 fatty acids help protect against heart disease.

Whole grains have a wealth of health benefits. Repeated studies have shown that the incidence of stroke, heart disease, and Type 2 diabetes are reduced due, in part, to the high levels of dietary fibre. The chances of asthma, high blood pressure, and inflammatory diseases could also be reduced.

Examples of whole grains are brown rice, oatmeal (not instant), and whole cornmeal.

Whole grains also provide important nutrients like:

- Folic acid to aid in red blood cell formation.
- Iron to help carry oxygen through the blood stream.
- B vitamins that help regulate metabolism.

- Selenium which is needed optimize your immune system.

Fruit is an essential part of getting the right amount of fibre and vitamins you need.

The suggested daily intake is about 2 servings. To optimize your intake, stay away from fruit juices as they have extra sugar and will make your blood sugar spike.

Eat strawberries, blueberries, apples, raspberries, oranges, or anything else you love.

Canned fruit is also fine, but make sure it is not packaged in syrup and has no added sugar.

Benefits of fruits are:

- Anti-oxidant properties for healthy skin and slower aging.
- Removal of free radicals.
- Vitamin A which is essential for eye health and protection from certain cancers.
- Vitamin C to protect against infections and improve iron absorption

Vegetables of all kinds are great for your health.

Some of the most advantageous are dark leafy greens which are a great source of anti-oxidants.

Yellow and orange vegetables like bell peppers, carrots, and summer squash contain high levels of vitamin C.

Eat at least two cups of vegetables a day.

Eating them raw, blanched, or steamed are the best ways to retain their health benefits.

Benefits of vegetables are:

- Great source of dietary fibre.
- Vitamin C for protection against flu and flu-like illnesses.
- Vitamin A for healthy mucous membranes.
- Vitamin K which limits neuronal damage in the brain.

Calcium is a very important component to help maintain bone strength and density. As you age, you are at a higher risk of osteoporosis. Calcium from various sources helps to delay the onset or prevent it all together. Calcium comes from dairy, of course, but you also have other options. This is especially helpful if you are lactose intolerant.

Great sources of Calcium include:

- Dairy like milk, cheese, and yogurt.
- Leafy greens including kale and spinach.
- Oranges.
- Salmon and sardines.
- Certain legumes like black beans, peas, and peanuts.

"Good" fats are important to your overall health. These include monounsaturated and polyunsaturated fats. Benefits of unsaturated fats eaten in moderation (less than 20% of your daily calorie needs) include improvements in blood sugar control and cholesterol levels, as well as protect against heart disease and lower blood pressure.

Sources of unsaturated fats include:

- Peanut butter.

- Fatty fish like trout, tuna, and salmon.
- Soymilk
- Avocados
- Nuts like cashews, almonds, and pecans.

Interesting Fact:

Unsaturated fats tend to be liquid at room temperature while saturated and trans fats are normally solid. Unsaturated oils like olive oil, sunflower oil, peanut oil, and canola oil are all good for you when used sparingly.

Good Health for a Long Life

Eating a healthy diet and taking the time to exercise offers so many benefits that doing it is a no-brainer.

The physical and mental health benefits of regular exercise are numerous, making you feel better, function better, and improve your outlook on life.

Eating the optimum amounts of fruit, vegetables, whole grain, dairy and unsaturated fats will improve your health from the inside out.

You could lower your blood pressure, lower the chance of developing Type 2 Diabetes, and also reduce your risk of heart disease.

Preparing healthy meals does not have to be a chore. There are many quick recipes for salads, soups, and main courses that will satisfy any time limit or attention span.

Exercising increases strength, flexibility, and promotes good mental health. Blood circulation improves along with lung function, bone density, and muscle mass.

Exercising has been shown time and again to boost your mood, lower your anxiety, and create an all-over feeling of well-being.

Healthy Eating

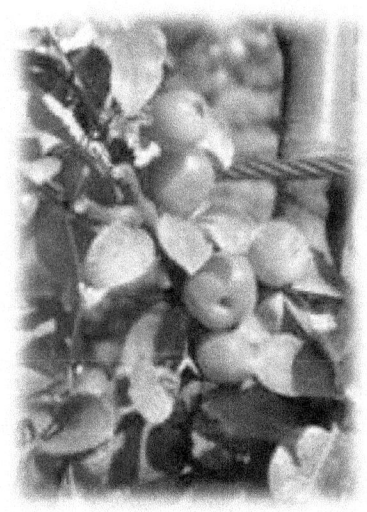

The way we eat today has evolved over the past few hundred years or so.

Not so much the content of our diet, but the way we choose and prepare our food.

If we had been living thousands of years ago, in pre-historic times when healthy eating was the only way available, we would probably have been eating meat and vegetables just as we do today.

However, the food didn't have lots of unhealthy ingredients added before being cooked to death and it certainly wasn't frozen for months and then 'nuked' in the microwave.

Our bodies weren't designed to eat a lot of the things that we eat today and we definitely weren't designed to consume preservatives, 'E' numbers and the other additives we find in processed food.

Our quest for convenience and simplicity has changed things drastically.

These days, when we go shopping, we look in the frozen section for things to put in our home freezer; then off to the pre-prepared vegetable section and dessert shelves so we can put together a meal for our family in record time.

Have you actually read what is contained in a simple can of baked beans that are labelled 'Healthy Living'? It contains – beans, tomatoes, water, sugar, modified cornflour, salt, seasoning, vinegar, flavouring and sweetener (saccharin).

I don't know about you, but if I see something that is labelled as 'healthy living' I would expect to see less of the additives. I'd like to bet that, in the days of cowboys out on the range, their baked beans didn't contain all these added extras…

Healthy eating does require a little more forward planning and effort than convenience living. But, ask yourself; is your overall health and well-being worth the extra effort?

Yes, of course it is.

Below are a few very simple rules to start you on your way to healthy eating

- Buy organic meat, vegetables, eggs, fruit etc. whenever you can. If the cost of organic produce is a problem, the next best thing is the 'free range' option for meat and eggs, and the freshest fruit and vegetables you can buy.

- Eat little and often – 5 small meals daily is much better for your system than 2 large meals.

- Learn to prepare and cook your food properly. Wash fruit and vegetables to remove any chemicals that may have been sprayed on them (unless they are organic) and trim excess fat from meat.

- Steam as much of your food as you can and avoid using fat in your cooking. You could also stir fry, grill and even boil. If you must boil vegetables however, don't boil them for very long as this will boil away the all the good vitamins that they contain.

- Eat as much raw food as you can. During cooking, food will lose of up to 97% of water-soluble vitamins A, D, E, and K.

- Avoid refined sugar as much as you can – use honey for sweetening.

- Avoid as much processed food as you possibly can – eat fresh whenever possible.

- Use lots of fresh herbs and spices in your cooking, avoiding salt as much as possible.

Make sure your healthy eating regime contains essential fatty acids. Studies have shown that low levels of essential fatty acids may be a factor in many modern illnesses. Some good sources of EFA are oily fish, seeds and leafy vegetables.

Healthy eating is all about balance and moderation.

Your body needs:

- Protein – provided by foods like beans, low-fat milk and meat.
- Carbohydrates – provided by such foods as whole grain breads and cereals, legumes, and starchy foods.
- A certain amount of 'good' fat.

As a general rule of thumb, the healthier fats are those which do not solidify at room temperature – olive oil, sunflower oil etc.

You also need an adequate supply of vitamins and minerals. So to ensure you get all these essential elements in your diet, you should eat healthy, balanced meals; cut out the fast food meals and highly processed foods and prepare your own food.

An added benefit of healthy eating is that you will probably lose those extra few pounds that have accumulated over the years – and without calorie counting.

How good is that?

Always eat a good breakfast containing complex carbohydrates to give you slow releasing energy which will help to avoid the drop in your blood sugar level mid-morning.

Try and have five small meals a day, eating small amounts of nutritious food at each meal means your body is always 'fuelled up'. Again, this will avoid your blood sugar dropping throughout the day.

Choose the healthy option when eating out – a good green salad with a juicy steak is always a favourite. Take your meals and snacks to work with you so you will always know what you are putting into your body.

Top Tip: *If you are making a sandwich and like butter on your bread, try using mayonnaise or salad cream instead of the butter. Butter has double the calories of mayonnaise and salad cream.*

Another great contribution to your new healthy eating regime would be to try juicing. (See later in the book for some great Juice recipes.)

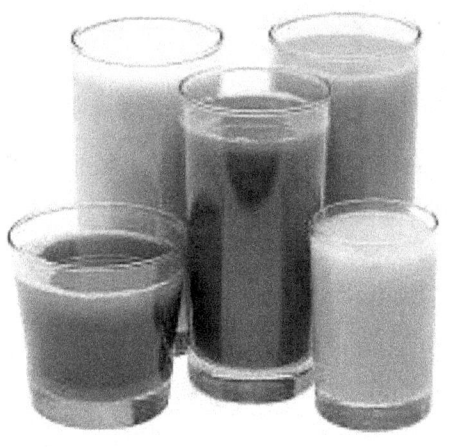

Although eating raw fruit and vegetables will provide substantial amounts of the vital nutrients they contain, much of the goodness is locked away in the fibre which is expelled from the body.

When you 'juice' fruit and vegetables, the goodness is released from the fibre so you can drink this highly concentrated liquid allowing the nutrients to be quickly absorbed into the bloodstream.

Our bodies will still need fibre which could be added to the juice in the form of flax seed or other dietary sources. Extra fibre could also be added to your meals in the form of vegetables etc.

Healthy eating is simple; you just need to make a conscious, informed choice when deciding what you eat or drink.

Moving from convenience food to fresh foods to help you to stay healthy will inevitably mean that you will be spending more time in the kitchen, but what price will you put on your own and your family's long term health?

Will it be worth it – of course it will.

Now, let's explore a little bit further.

A lot of the supermarket convenience foods are easy to prepare and cook. They are usually processed tins and packets, so you just need to open the packet or tin and pop it into the microwave, give it a quick 'nuke' and hey presto – dinner's ready.

That's OK if your only aim is to fill your stomach.

But have you given any thought as to why pre-packaged convenience foods are able to have such a long sell by date?

They keep for an un-naturally long time either in the cupboard or in the fridge without deteriorating because they are so deficient in living ingredients and so full of preservatives.

Natures 'Fast Food Restaurant'

Fast and convenient food is extremely popular in today's frantic lifestyles but have you ever stopped to think about the very first fast foods?

The very first fast foods were from nature's own larder.

Nature has provided us with all the fast foods we could want in the form of vegetables, fruit, nuts, berries, herbs and spring water etc. and a lot of this natural food is low in calories as well as being extremely good for us..

Ok, so the hunter gatherer gig is no longer the way to go, but consider how much healthier we would be if we were to return to the diet food that nature has provided for us.

Consider dining in Nature's Fast Food Restaurant occasionally.

Eat a meal that consists of the things that you could go out and gather yourself if you had the time (and inclination) to.

Have you ever thought how convenient these fruits, vegetables, berries and herbs are? They are mostly within the reach of an average adult human, and those that aren't easily reachable usually drop to the ground when they are ripe and ready to eat.

How convenient is that?

If you think it is time to make some changes in the way you eat, here are a few easy things to substitute to make your everyday diet just a little healthier.

- Instead of Sweet Fruit Yoghurts try Natural Yoghurt with fresh fruit added
- Instead of Ice Cream try Natural Yoghurt with fresh fruit, frozen
- Instead of Breakfast Cereals try Porridge Oats
- Instead of White Bread try Wholemeal Bread
- Instead of White Pasta try Wholemeal Pasta
- Instead of Whole Milk try Skimmed Milk
- Instead of Sweet Snacks try Vegetable or Fruit pieces
- Instead of Soda try Fresh Fruit Juice with added sparkling water

- Instead of Tea and Coffee try Herbal Teas or decaffeinated tea or coffee

Another great idea is to substitute at least one of your daily meals for raw foods – you can eat as much as you like as well. There are lots of things to choose from like raw bean-sprouts, peppers, courgette, lettuce, tomatoes, beetroot, apples, pears, cucumber, celery, carrot, and so on.

Top Tip: *Grate a selection of raw fruit and vegetables, combine in a large bowl and add a simple olive oil and lemon juice dressing – yummy.*

Eat your meals sitting at a table. If you eat 'on the run'; it will take your body longer to register the 'full' feeling in your brain and you end up eating much more than you intended.

Snack as often as you like with raw vegetables and fruit in order to avoid the drop in your blood sugar levels.

A Few Facts about Modern Fast Food Restaurants

No-one is saying that you should never have an occasional meal from one of the growing range of fast food restaurants. But, as in most things, moderation is the key. After reading the following facts, you will be able to make an informed decision and decide if it really is worth it.

McDonald's – A juicy hamburger with a side of fries sounds delicious. But if you take a regular Double Quarter Pound Cheeseburger with a side of medium sized fries you will be eating approximately 60g of fat and 1,100 calories total for the fries and the cheeseburger (not to mention whatever you wash it down with).

Kentucky Fried Chicken - Their chicken is a popular choice for a quick and easy meal. But one original recipe chicken breast is approximately 21g of fat and 360 calories. If you have 2 chicken breasts from one of their popular family bucket meals, you're looking at 42g of fat and 720 calories. This doesn't include any side dishes that might come with the meal, such as fries, coleslaw, or beans.

Pizza Hut Pizza – It's so easy to come home exhausted and fall prey to the convenience of pizza delivery. A Large Pepperoni pan pizza has about 14g of total fat and 270 total calories **per slice**. If you eat 2 slices of that pizza, you will have consumed around 28g of fat and about 540 calories total. Add extra cheese or other toppings and you'll cost yourself even more fat and calories.

Subway – You think you're eating healthy, but it depends on what menu item you choose. A 6" Chicken Parmesan sandwich is approximately 18g of fat and around 500 calories. This doesn't include any sides. If you add more sauce to your sandwich, you'll need to figure more calories into the equation.

Choosing Healthy Food from the Supermarket

If you are trying to shed a few pounds, do you search for the latest fat free products on the supermarket shelves and load your shopping cart with every one?

Well, did you know that just because the label says 'fat free' or 'low fat' does not necessarily mean that the product is low in calories? Remember when you are shopping for healthy food that fat free does not always mean non-fattening. Check labels if you are unsure.

Better still, try and avoid all processed food and eat freshly prepared meat and vegetables.

When you go shopping, always go *after* you have eaten, it is a well-known fact that shopping when you are hungry will encourage you to buy the wrong type of foods. You will also buy more when you are hungry, so eating before you shop can also save you money.

Before you go shopping, make a list and stick to it; avoid the temptation of impulse buying.

When you are trying to improve your health and lose a few pounds, try and think of solutions so that you are not denying yourself the stuff that you like.

For instance, if you love bread, look for the wholegrain option or if you can't possibly live without chocolate, buy a bar and allow yourself two squares every day.

Alternatively, you could have one day a week where you can choose to eat whatever takes your fancy. As long as you return to the healthy eating, it will certainly not ruin your weight loss and health maintenance plans.

Drink as much water as you can to keep you hydrated. The more water you can drink, the better it is for you. Our body can go for weeks without food but without water your organs would very soon begin to fail and before a week is up you would most probably be dead.

Buy a smaller dinner plate. If you usually use a 12" plate, buy a 9" one. You will not feel deprived when you see a full plate rather than a smaller portion on your usual dinner plate.

By changing just a few things in your lifestyle you could end up looking and feeling fantastic without feeling deprived of anything that you like. That has got to be good.

If you just change your eating habits a little at a time, you will soon begin to notice the pounds melting away, your skin will be better, your energy levels will increase etc. and all without a great deal of effort.

It is not difficult to make healthy meals that are good for your mind, heart, and body. The perception is that using fresh, non-processed ingredients is going to turn meal preparation into some kind of marathon event.

It doesn't have to be that way.

Instead, use simple ingredients that are quick and easy to put together. Spending an extra fifteen minutes making a fresh and nutritious meal will be well worth it – and you know exactly what you are eating.

So, to summarize, you don't have to be a college professor to learn about and practise leading a healthy lifestyle. You just have to be aware of the improvements you need to make to remain as fit and healthy as you can as you approach old age.

A Few Simple Recipe Suggestions

These recipes are suggested because most of them allow you to use your personal favourite ingredients to make a meal that you know you will enjoy. After all, what's the point in cooking if you are not sure that you will like the meal?

Breakfast

You should always eat breakfast. It jump starts your body's metabolism after a night of rest. If you're not a morning person and often don't have time to make breakfast, combine yogurt, granola, and fresh blackberries, a banana or raspberries for a quick meal.

Make your own Muesli

Get an airtight container, a pack of organic oats, dried fruit and nuts of your preference, some bran, linseed and any other ingredients that you like.

Fill the container to half with oats, add bran and linseed; shake up to mix well. Next add a selection of your choice of dried fruit and nuts then shake to combine all the ingredients.

Hey presto, healthy breakfast with no waste - because you chose all the ingredients that you like.

Try a Glass of Kefir for Breakfast.

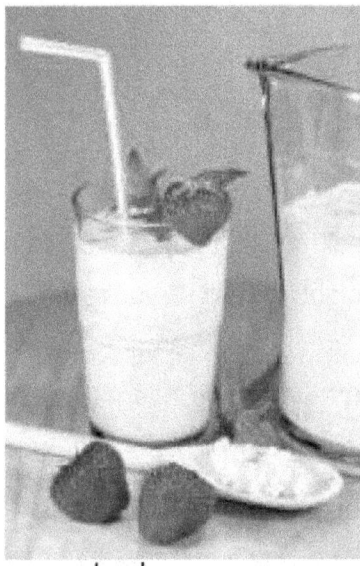

"What is Kefir?" I hear you ask.

Well, Kefir is a cultured milk drink that is made using 'grains' of Kefir.

Kefir is a cultured, enzyme-rich food filled with friendly micro-organisms that help balance your 'inner ecosystem'.

Easily digested, it cleanses the intestines, provides beneficial bacteria and yeast, vitamins and minerals, and complete proteins.

More nutritious and therapeutic than yoghurt, it supplies complete protein, essential minerals, and valuable B vitamins that are essential to us all.

Kefir is rich in Vitamin B12, B1, and Vitamin K. It is an excellent source of biotin, a B Vitamin which aids the body's assimilation of other B Vitamins, such as folic acid, pantothenic acid, and B12.

The numerous benefits of maintaining adequate B vitamin intake range from regulation of the kidneys, liver and nervous system to helping relieve skin disorders, boost energy, the immune system and it promotes longevity.

In order to make Kefir you will need a starter community of Kefir grains which are added to the liquid you wish to ferment – usually organic milk.

Kefir grains cannot be produced from scratch, but the grains grow during fermentation, and additional grains are produced.

Kefir grains can be bought from other growers.

I bought my first grains on Ebay and have since supplied lots of other people as my grains grew. A starter community of Kefir grains is not expensive and can last for a number of years as they increase in size.

You can freeze or dry the surplus grains to save for future use. Or share them with family and friends.

If you have any trouble getting a starter community of Kefir grains and would like to give it a try, send me an email (address at end of book) and, if I have any available, I will send you some to get you started for the price of postage. (Please bear in mind that I live in UK)

Some people (me included...) find the sharp taste of Kefir not to their taste. My solution is to add a banana and honey to the milk and blend to a lovely refreshing breakfast shake.

Any soft fruit could be used or even just honey to sweeten the Kefir. You could even add a spoonful of peanut butter to your Kefir before blending. I have a half pint glass of banana and honey Kefir each morning – it is delicious.

Experiment with different flavours – you can find lots of different recipes online plus a lot of information on the benefits of Kefir for health and longevity.

Porridge

Porridge is a great way to start the day. If you prefer your porridge to be sweetened, use honey rather than sugar. Another way to jazz up a bowl of this nutritious breakfast is to add some fruit. Strawberries, raspberries, blueberries, bananas etc. all make a good bowl of porridge great.

Traditional Fry-Up

If you cannot imagine life without a traditional fry-up you don't need to give it up. Simply change the way you cook it. Grill the bacon, sausage and tomato and scramble or poach the eggs. Even small changes like that can drastically reduce the amount of fat that you eat.

Eggs

If you love the idea for eggs for breakfast, try this easy way of preparing them.

Preheat the oven to 180°. Take an ovenproof ramekin and add a little sunflower oil to the bottom.

Wipe the oil all over the dish using a piece of kitchen paper then put in the oven for 2 minutes. Break two eggs into the already warm dish and season with salt and pepper. Put in oven for about 6 minutes and when nearly done take out and sprinkle with a little grated cheese. Return to oven until cheese is melted and golden brown. Serve with a slice of really fresh wholemeal bread.

Is there a better way to start the day?

Fruit Breakfast

A lovely way to start the day is with a bowl of fresh fruit.

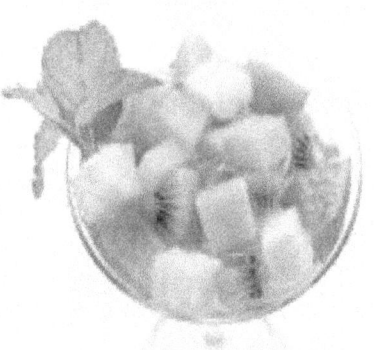

Prepare your fruit half an hour before you need it and refrigerate. Cold fruit really does taste so much better.

Use kiwi, papaya, mango, grapes, pineapple etc. to bring the taste of summer to your day.

No need to add anything unless you prefer a little natural yoghurt to add to the flavours.

Bread

If, like me, you are a lover of bread, try a plate of different types of bread spread with a reduced sugar jam or even just a spoon of honey. You could have any of a wide variety of bread that is available these days. Bagels, soda bread, flat breads, walnut and raisin, sundried tomato, etc. etc. the list is huge…

Juice

For a refreshing, quick and healthy way to start the day, try one of the juice recipes included in this book.

Lunch

If you have lunch at work, take your own rather than buy a snack from the shop so you will always know exactly what you are eating. You can be imaginative when you pack up your lunch. Remember to add a few extras to snack on throughout the day.

Buy one of the oil sprays and use when frying, at just one calorie per spray it takes the guilt out of frying food.

Mediterranean Salad

Use precooked whole grain pasta stored in a zip lock bag in the refrigerator. Turn that into a wonderful Mediterranean pasta salad without having to wait for the pasta to chill. Cut up tomatoes, spring onions, peppers, add olives, pour a balsamic vinaigrette over it and you're done.

Fish

Salmon and other fish are fast and easy to bake. While you're waiting for the oven to preheat, boil two pans of water, one for couscous, rice or pasta and the other for broccoli. The couscous, rice or pasta goes in first, the fish goes into the oven next, and the broccoli is boiled until it's a healthy green colour. Making a lunch like this takes 20 minutes, tops.

Chicken

Take a cooked chicken breast; add a large green salad and a simple olive oil and lemon dressing for a delicious summer lunch. Serve with chunks of very fresh bread.

Tuna

Combine a can of tuna with cooked basmati rice, diced peppers and corn, add lemon juice, finely chopped chilli and fresh herbs. This is a great lunch – hot or cold. You can substitute the rice for cooked pasta if you prefer. Serve with tortilla wraps.

Dinner

Top Tip: Don't eat dinner after 9pm; give your body time to digest the food before going to bed.

Jacket Potato

Prick a large potato all over and put in the oven to bake. Serve with a large salad and your choice of filling.

Homemade Vegetable Soup

Choose a selection of your favourite vegetables, peel and cut into chunks. Cook in a chicken or vegetable stock. When the vegetables are soft remove from heat and leave to cool slightly. Remove a cup or two of the vegetables and blitz the remainder in a blender being very careful not to overfill it. Blitz the soup in batches if you need to.

Return the blitzed soup to the saucepan and add the vegetables that you removed earlier. Taste and adjust seasoning if necessary. Reheat when required.

Serve with fresh crusty bread.

Crab Cakes

You will need a tin of crab meat, a few chopped spring onions, a clove of garlic, chopped chilli, grated courgette and red pepper, well dried, and beaten egg to bind the mixture together. You could create your own ingredient list using whatever fish or grated vegetables you prefer.

Combine all the ingredients well and form into small round shapes. Fry in a non-stick pan with a spray of oil.

Serve with boiled new potatoes tossed in mint and a selection of vegetables or a green salad.

Burger and Fries

Buy some very lean minced beef; add finely chopped onion, very finely chopped chilli, and a selection of your favourite finely chopped vegetables. Mix together thoroughly using a beaten egg to bind if necessary and form into small circles.

You could choose to oven cook or fry in a non-stick pan sprayed with oil.

To make the fries:

Take and peel a large potato. Cut into thick strips then boil in lightly salted water until just beginning to soften. Drain well on kitchen paper; then place in a single layer onto a baking tray and spray with oil.

Bake in a hot oven until golden brown turning the fries to ensure that they brown evenly.

Spinach Stuffed Chicken

Split a skinned chicken breast carefully to make a pocket. Place a very large handful of spinach and a crushed clove of garlic in a pan with a the juice of half a lemon.

Cook over a medium heat until spinach is just beginning to wilt. Remove from heat and stir in some grated parmesan cheese. Add freshly ground black pepper.

Stuff your chicken breast with the spinach and cheese mixture. Wrap the whole thing tightly with a rasher of lean bacon using a skewer to keep it together.

Place in an ovenproof dish, cover and bake in a moderate oven.

Serve with new potatoes tossed in finely chopped chives or a fresh green salad.

Tip: You can use any cooked vegetables or herbs to fill your chicken breast.

Juicing and Smoothies

Juicing is a great way to add essential vitamins and minerals to your daily diet. It is also a good way to encourage children to eat fruit and vegetables that they wouldn't normally eat.

For smoothies you will need a food blender._For the juicing you will need a juicing machine. Don't start out with an expensive state of the art machine; try a cheap and cheerful one until you are confident that juicing will become part of your daily life.

TOP TIP: *If you are not sure about the savoury taste of some of the vegetable juices, try adding an apple to the ingredients. As well as adding a little sweetness to your juice, you also benefit from adding yet another ingredient to your juice.*

Below are some simple combinations you can try.

But the fun of juicing and smoothie making is devising your own combinations.

2 large carrots

Large handful of spinach

1 avocado

1 apple

––––––––––––––

2 thick slices of pineapple

1 mango

1 mashed banana (You could add milk to this for a refreshing smoothie.)

––––––––––––––

1 apple

2 large carrots

Quarter of a raw beetroot

A small piece of ginger.

––––––––––––––

½ lettuce

2 apples

½ mango

_____

1 beetroot

1 apple

2 sticks celery

Handful of spinach

_____

25 Health & Fitness Facts

- **Exercise.** When you exercise your brain releases the chemicals serotonin and dopamine. These are what make us feel calm, happy, and euphoric. The extra oxygen taken in can also improve mental clarity and thinking.

- **Weight-bearing** Exercise. Walking, jogging, dancing or lifting weights, strengthens bone formation and helps prevent osteoporosis in later life. And it isn't just women who suffer from this; men can be just as at risk.

- **Regular Physical Exercise.** Will strengthen your heart and make it pump blood more efficiently. If your heart can work less to pump the blood around your body, the force on your arteries decreases, lowering your blood pressure. By lowering blood pressure and improving circulation, exercise can help to prevent heart disease. Gentle exercise can also strengthen the heart after a heart attack and help prevent further problems.

- **Lungs.** As you exercise you take more air into your lungs in order to get the extra oxygen to your cells. The more regularly you exercise the stronger and more efficient your lungs will be. The oxygen you take in when exercising can be over double that of the intake when you are sedentary.

- **Healthy Diet.** Exercise combined with a healthy diet that includes plenty of fruit and veg, whole grains and fish will help you to lose any extra pounds, tone up muscles and give you a leaner version of you.

- **Diet.** Whole grains are excellent sources of fibre and other important nutrients, such as selenium, potassium and magnesium. They have been linked to a lower risk of heart disease, diabetes and certain cancers. Because they're metabolised quicker they give you more sustainable energy release keeping you going for longer.

- **Fish**. Fish is full of essential fats, which is good news for your heart, brain and arteries. You also get a healthy dose of calcium which is beneficial for your bones and better muscle function. So include fish, such as salmon, fresh tuna and mackerel, at least twice a week.

- **Always eat Breakfast**. Breakfast refuels you and sets you up for the day. Without it you can get tired, restless and irritable. Researchers believe that eating first thing in the morning may help to stabilise blood sugar levels, which regulate appetite and energy. And starting the day with those all-important whole grains will mean you are raring to go.

- **Stop Smoking.** It goes without saying that you should stop smoking. There are over 4000 compounds in a single cigarette, many are toxic, meaning they damage your cells, and a fair amount are carcinogenic which means they are cancer causing. So if you smoke the best thing you can do for your body today is to stop.

- **Walk.** There is nothing better than walking. Walking a mile every day promises to reduce the risk of heart disease as well as strengthen your bones and keep them strong. Walking is free and easy to slot into your life. Two 15 minute walks a day will have a noticeable, positive effect on your life.

- **Fun Exercise.** Find something you enjoy. Getting fit doesn't have to mean gruelling workouts at the gym, pounding the pavements for hours on end or struggling to keep up in a fitness class. Any type of exercise that causes you to sweat and increase your heart rate is good for you. Try a few different things and find something you enjoy.

- **Spot Reduction.** There is no such thing as spot reduction. If you have a flabby overhang no amount of crunches will turn that into a 6 pack if you don't also lose the fat. A well rounded fitness regime will take in cardio activity, weight bearing and flexibility. Swimming is excellent for combining all three.

- **Help Hold Back the Years.** Research into telerome length, (the protective ends of your chromosomes that shorten as you age), has shown that regular exercise stops the teleromes from shortening. This helps you ward off age related illness and stay healthier and active for longer, which will prolong life expectancy and life quality.

- **Make it a Priority for YOU.** It's sometimes very hard to start an exercise programme. Life has a way of intruding and everything else always seems to take priority. It is important though that you take the time to incorporate some fitness into your routine. Pick a time when you feel it would be best for you and allocate that time. Let others know that this is what will be happening. The fitter you are the better you will function, so those little slots of time that you devote to yourself will have a major impact on other areas of your life.
- **Good Fitness Levels = Good Immunity.** As well as warding off disease such as heart disease, stroke and Type 2 Diabetes, regular exercise will also help protect you against those day-to-day illnesses such as the common cold or flu and can even help you recover faster from a minor infection. So don't stop exercising just because you are a little bit under the weather. (Although always check with a doctor regarding long-term or chronic illness).
- **Back Pain**. About 8 in every 10 people will suffer with some type of back pain. Back pain can be

managed or prevented with a fitness program that includes muscle strengthening and flexibility. Having good posture and a strong abdomen is the body's best defence against back pain.

- **Self Esteem.** Improved self-esteem is one of the top benefits of regular physical activity. While exercising, your body releases chemicals called endorphins that can improve your mood and the way you feel about yourself. The feeling that follows a run or workout is often described as "euphoric". Exercise can help you cope with stress and ward off depression and anxiety.

- **Stress Relief.** In small doses stress is good for us because it's a motivator. However chronic or long term stress is very damaging. Exercise relieves stress in several ways. Cardio workouts stimulate brain chemicals that encourage growth of nerve cells. Exercise increases the activity of serotonin and dopamine. And lastly, a raised heart rate releases endorphins and a hormone known as ANP, which reduces pain, induces euphoria, and helps control the brain's response to stress and anxiety. A brisk walk in the park will do this as effectively as a fast paced gym session.

- **Raise your Heartbeat.** You can reap all the physical and mental health benefits of exercise with 30 minutes of moderate exercise four times a week. Two 15 minute exercise sessions can also work just as well. So utilise all those little spare chunks of time in the day to think about spending 15 minutes raising your heart rate.
- **S.M.A.R.T.** Repeatedly failing to stick to your goals means that either your goal is out of reach or that you haven't quite established what to do to reach it. Think S.M.A.R.T. Make your goals:
  - Specific
  - Measurable
  - Attainable
  - Realistic
  - Targeted.

So rather than the goal to 'get fit', find a way to break it down into realistic chunks. For instance: 'I will go for a brisk walk/jog three times a week'. By giving yourself something specific to work towards the whole goal of 'get fit' won't seem so daunting.

- **Relax**. Let it become part of your life rather than a chore. By thinking of fitness as a lifestyle choice rather than a task that has to be ticked off it will be easier to incorporate it into your daily life. Activities with the children or friends, vigorous housework and when you're on the go will all present opportunities to be more active.

- **Variety.** While all exercise has enormous health benefits it is good to get in a mix of cardio, strength & flexibility. Aerobic activities such as running, cycling, and swimming strengthen your heart and increase your endurance.

- **Avoid Frailty**. Strength training such as weight lifting or resistance training builds muscle and bone mass, improves balance and could help prevent falls. It's one of the best ways to help avoid frailty in old age. Flexibility exercises such as stretching and yoga help prevent injury, enhance range of motion, reduce stiffness, and limit aches and pains.

- **Sleep.** If may not seem obvious but sleep is important for overall health. It involves two hormones, leptin and ghrelin. These two hormones work together to control our feeling of hunger and fullness. Lack of sleep drives leptin levels down and it causes ghrelin levels to rise. So this means that the next day after you have not had enough sleep you will feel hungrier and you will not feel full after eating.

- **Moderate Exercise.** Many people starting out on a new fitness regime are confused by the term moderate exercise. Injury can be caused by overdoing it at the beginning. So for clarification, moderate exercise means that you breathe a little heavier than normal, but are not out of breath and that your body feels warmer as you move, but not overheated or very sweaty.

Motivation

We know physical exercise benefits us in many ways. Yet, we are still searching for a very good reason to begin and then even more reasons to continue.

Is this you?

- Buy the next 'best thing' in exercise DVDs. Watch them through a couple of times then put them with all the others to begin later...

- Join the gym, buying the full year's subscription; reasoning that it will encourage you to attend regularly. Start with enthusiasm, going twice a week and telling everyone. Then you begin to find reasons that you can't go this week...

- Decide to train for the next big city marathon. Jog to work twice a week. Then decide that you don't have enough time to do the training. So back to the car...

- Buy a Wii-Fit, try it once and put it back in the box for next week...

We know that regular exercise greatly benefits our health. It strengthens the bones, cartilage, spinal column, nervous system, muscles and joints.

Exercise is a great way to help reduce risks of strokes, heart disease, diabetes, high-blood pressure, high cholesterol etc. We also know that we will feel better about ourselves when we've managed to lose some of the fat that we've built up over the years.

Remember, fat is like wearing a jacket – to see the body properly, first you have to take it off.

However, what most of us lack is the *motivation* to sustain a regular health and exercise plan.

7 Ways to Sustain the Good Intentions

1. Measure, weigh and take a photo of yourself before you begin your new routine.
2. Stick your photo up where you can see it. If you would rather no-one else saw it, stick it up on the inside of the cupboard door.
3. Get your children, grandchildren, best friend or partner involved or all of them. You're doing

something that will be good for everyone so you can motivate each other.

4. Choose something FUN to do. Try 20 minutes football in the park, power walking (who cares if you look silly – wiggle that behind…), cycling or, in bad weather get out that Wii-Fit and have some fun.

5. Set your exercise for a regular time each week or day or whatever. Stick your agreed schedule on the fridge door. If children are involved, you can be sure they will not let you get out of your scheduled activity.

6. Only weigh yourself once a fortnight or, even better, once a month. Throw out the bathroom scales to avoid the temptation.

7. Take a new photo each month and stick it up next to the older photos. You will be able to see the physical changes as each new photo is put up.

Each have a turn at deciding what activities to do and have a go at anything that is suggested, even if the young ones want to play skipping or chasing – at least give it your best shot. As long as it involves some physical exercise that increases your heart rate, you will reap the benefits – I guarantee it.

Now, what are you waiting for – go and recruit your motivators.

A Healthy Mind

As we get older, maintaining a healthy mind is just as important as maintaining a healthy body.

Being 'old' is as much a state of mind as it is about your fitness.

It's not much good being in tiptop physical condition if we don't intend to enjoy life.

It's time to become a 'glass half full' type of person.

Tips to Lift Your Mood

For a few simple tips to lift your mood, please read on:

One of the first things to observe is how you form your sentences. What words do you use when you are speaking and even when you are thinking?

Are your words negative with lots of 'don't' and 'can't'?

By using 'can't' and 'don't' in your everyday language, you are focusing on the negative, which is what you don't want to happen. Instead, try reinforcing the positive, which is what you *do* want to happen.

For example:

Don't forget	becomes	Remember to…
Don't panic	becomes	Stay calm
Don't be late	becomes	Please be on time
I don't know how to…	becomes	I can/will learn how to
I can't find…	becomes	It will turn up

You get the idea…

It would be very difficult to monitor all your thoughts and words – that would be a very daunting task; but you can observe how you are feeling (your mood). Our moods give us a very clear indication of our thought pattern.

For example; it is very difficult to be in a joyful mood and think negative thoughts. On the other hand, you would find it difficult to be depressed and think positive thoughts.

Once you are able to recognise how your mind is working, you will find it easier to do something about it.

But do remember, you can't jump from feeling utterly miserable to feeling ecstatic in one leap. You should aim for a slightly better feeling thought, then the next slightly better feeling thought and so on…

When you notice that your words and thoughts are becoming negative, you know; the sad, doom and gloom type. You could put on your favourite upbeat or relaxing music – whatever works for you, sing along or just sit and close your eyes, smile (it's really hard to be miserable when you are smiling…) and really concentrate on the music and the *really good things* in your life for a while.

If you are in a place where you are struggling to find really good things to think about, consider these:

- You are alive and breathing
- You have some great music to listen to
- You have a roof over your head
- You have some great friends and family

You could spend a few minutes writing down all the things that you are grateful for.

Why should the simple act of thinking about and acknowledging who and what you are grateful for, make such a big difference in your life?

Here are just a few reasons:

- **Because it reminds you of the positive things in your life**. It helps you appreciate the people in your life; whether they're loved ones or just a stranger you met who was kind to you in some way.

- **Because it turns bad things into good things**. Having problems at work? Be grateful you have work. Be grateful you have challenges, and that life isn't boring. Be grateful that you can learn from these challenges. Be thankful they make you a stronger person.

- **Because it reminds you of what's important**. It's hard to complain about the little things when you give thanks that your children are alive and healthy. It's hard to get stressed out over paying bills when you are grateful there is a roof over your head.

- **Because it reminds you to thank others**. The simple act of saying "thank you" to someone can make a big difference in that person's life. Calling them, emailing them, stopping by to say thank you - just taking that minute out of your life to tell them why you are grateful toward them is important to them. People like being appreciated for who they are and what they do. It costs you little, but makes someone else happy. And making someone else happy will make you happy.

So, find a place where you won't be disturbed and sit quietly and reflect on the reasons you have to be grateful.

Maybe set your alarm for 30 minutes earlier or you could even pull over in a beautiful parking spot to get those few minutes to yourself.

Show your gratitude every day and you'll find your life being filled with more and more things to be grateful for.

Now, don't you feel just a little bit better?

Then you could have a soak in the bath whilst reading your favourite book. I bet you will feel better still.

Reading a good book is a great way to take you into another world which helps to diminish your depression or worries.

You could go to the gym, or for a long walk with the dog whilst listening to some great music or inspirational stuff on your MP3 player. Now can you feel your mood lifting?

When you feel your mood is not as 'upbeat' as you would like, choose an activity that makes you concentrate on something other than yourself and your problems.

Dwelling on a problem will not help you to solve it; it simply magnifies it in your mind. Tell yourself that the solution will come to you – and believe it.

Smile – it's hard to feel miserable when you are smiling.

Remember the objective, to feel just a little bit better – one step at a time.

If you find yourself feeling a bit down just before bedtime, have a warm bath. This washes away all the negative energies that you have picked up during the day. Add some lavender essential oil and relax for ten minutes.

When you get into bed, spend a few minutes thinking about all the good things in your life and how tomorrow will bring great things. Lots of positive thoughts.

This helps your subconscious mind to assimilate everything you need for a great day when you wake up.

~~~~~~~~~~~~~~~~

Make a commitment to yourself to improve your health and your mind. The benefit isn't just for you, but for your children and grandchildren.

You won't have to miss a thing.

Start today, don't leave it until tomorrow, next week, or when you have the time – just do it.

Contact me:

If you would like to be notified of the release of the next book in this series, please send an email to:

info@uk-digitalmedia.co.uk

You can also use this email address to request a starter community of Kefir grains.

DISCLAIMER

All information in the book is for general information purposes only.

The author has used her best efforts in preparing this information and makes no representations or warranties with respect to the accuracy, applicability or completeness of the material contained within.

Furthermore, the author takes no responsibility for any errors, omissions or inaccuracies in this document. The author disclaims any implied or expressed warranties or fitness for any particular purpose.

The author shall in no event be held liable for losses or damages whatsoever. The author assumes no responsibility or liability for any consequences resulting directly or indirectly from any action or lack of action that you take based on the information in this document.

Use of the publication and suggestions therein is at your own risk.

This document is not medical advice and should not be treated as such. Always consult your doctor for medical advice before starting any diet or exercise program.

This book is not a substitute for medical advice and treatment. The author is not a health professional and urges you to seek professional medical advice if you have or suspect you have a health problem. Results will vary depending on your circumstances and no warranties or representations are made with respect to your own results.

Reproduction or translation of any part of this publication by any means, electronic or mechanical, without the permission of the author, is both forbidden and illegal. You are not permitted to share, sell, and trade or give away this document and it is for your own personal use only, unless stated otherwise. Each document may be marked with an invisible watermark to allow the author to identify the original customer of the document.

By using any of the suggestions in this publication, you agree that you have read the disclaimer and agree with all the terms.